Copyright© 2019 Rainey Leigh Seraphine
Wizzenhill Publishing

All rights reserved. Without limiting the rights under copyright reserved above, no part of this work/publication may be reproduced, stored in or introduced into a retrieval system, or transmitted, in any form or by any means (electronic, mechanical, print, photocopying, recording or otherwise) without the prior written permission of the copyright owner.

ISBN 978-0-6485458-3-5

For Theo
and all the little people
whose worlds
are as big as his

Theo's World

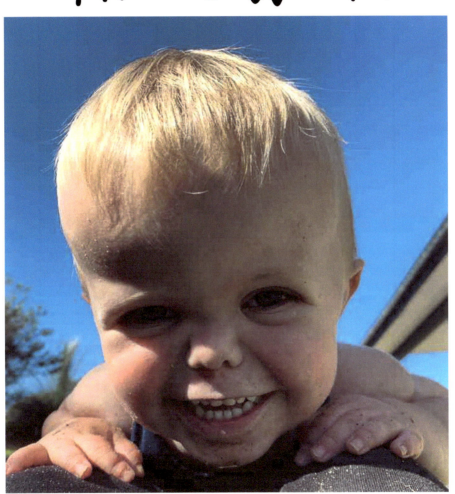

A few thoughts from Karina, Theo's Mum

I would like to be honest and although I find it hard to put into words, I'll give it a go.

The joy of Theo's birth was overshadowed when we found out he was born with dwarfism. It was hard to deal with, hard to comprehend. To be honest, I'm still ashamed of how I reacted. The feelings were completely unexpected and I didn't know how to cope with them at first.

You still love, with all of your heart, the tiny baby that you have created, but you worry about the life they will have, the way they will be treated, and what complications will come their way.

You see other kids their age doing things that your child should be doing and it is hard. You grieve for the life you thought your child would have. Although I'm happy he won't be playing football!

And then, amongst the worries, you watch them reach their own special milestones and you're filled with precious joy.

All you want is for your child to be healthy and happy. Dwarfism has many ongoing complications and you dearly hope that your child doesn't suffer too much. It's never easy watching your child go under anaesthetic. Throughout Theo's early years, there have been frequent hospital visits and I'm very thankful for the amazing specialists and the public health system.

There is a long road ahead. Theo has just turned three. In spite of the worries, I wouldn't change him having dwarfism. He wouldn't be Theo any other way. He is so cheeky and funny already, and as you watch him, you just know he will be the life of the party because no one is going to knock him down.

It's time for the derogatory names, staring and bullying to stop. A person is a person no matter how small and I think the following pages will prove that our Theo is one heck of a worthy human being.

We love you Theo.

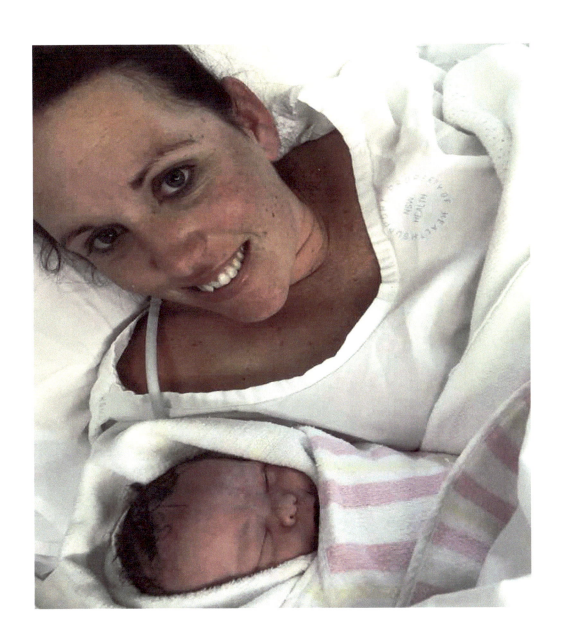

I am quite small
as you can see.
Smaller than most
in my world you'll agree.
I will never be tall,
although I will grow,
there's something inside me,
something I know.
Just like the Tardis,
of Dr Who,
I'm much bigger inside,
just like you.

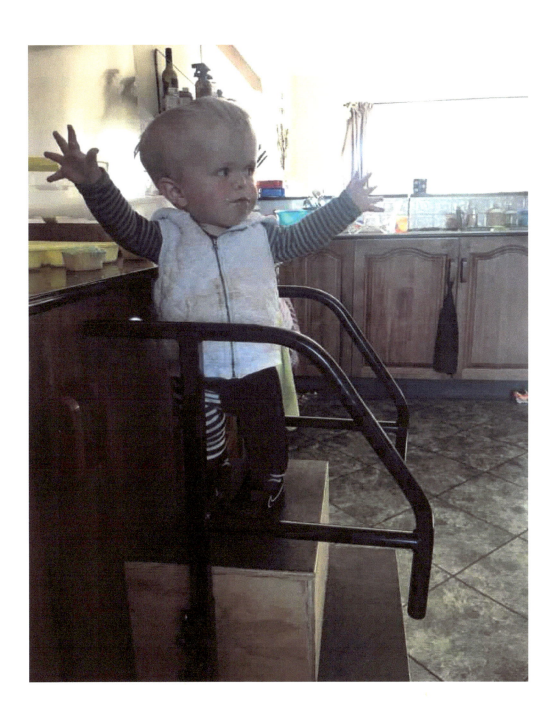

My head seems quite large,
I know it is true.
My arms are quite short,
and my legs are too.
It just seems the way
that it has to be,
but I really don't mind
'cause it's fun to be me.
My name is Theo,
and this is my world.
You'll see who I am
as my story unfurls.

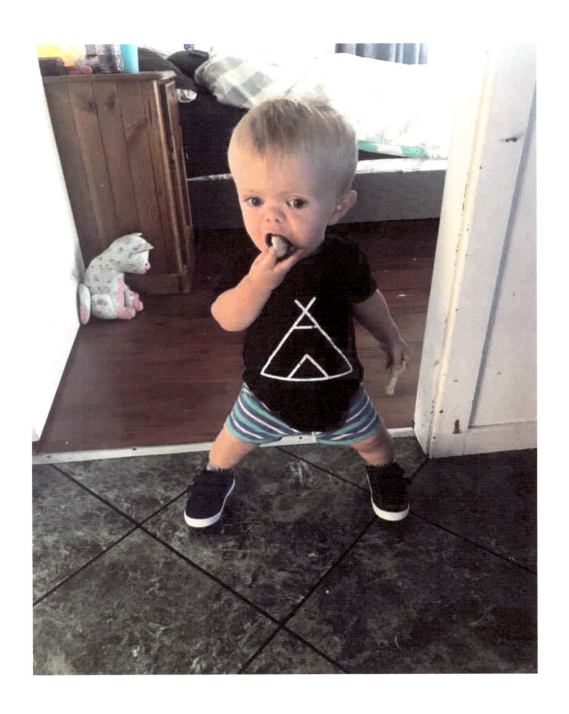

What is your favourite
thing that you do?
Is it playing on swings?
Hey, that is mine too.
Do you swing with your sister,
or brother or friends?
Hey, I love that too
as the fun never ends.
Except when Mum says
it's now time to stop,
so I swing one last time
before hopping off
and imagine I've reached
the tallest tree top.

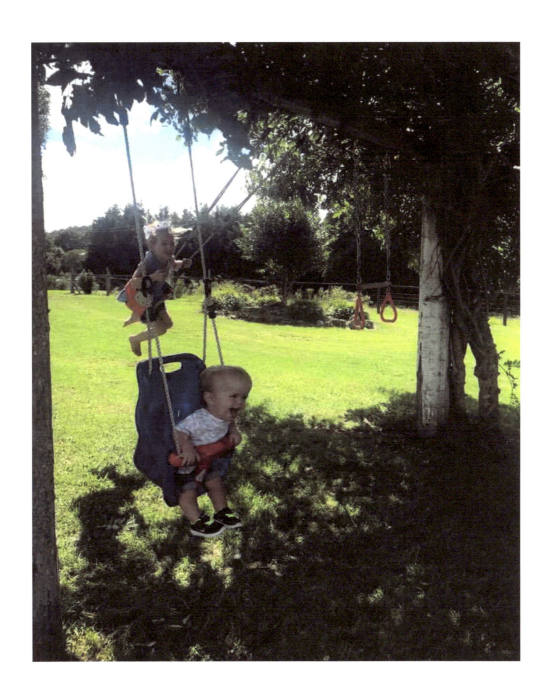

Perhaps you like puddles,
or playing in mud?
If you're somewhat like me
you have mud in your blood.
There is nothing so fine
as a good splash and splosh.
To throw heaps of pebbles
and cause heaps of plops.
To wriggle my legs,
hands and feet and my toes
and stick out my tongue
and wrinkle my nose.
Mud puddles are cool,
I think you'll agree.
Do you love them as much,
or more possibly?

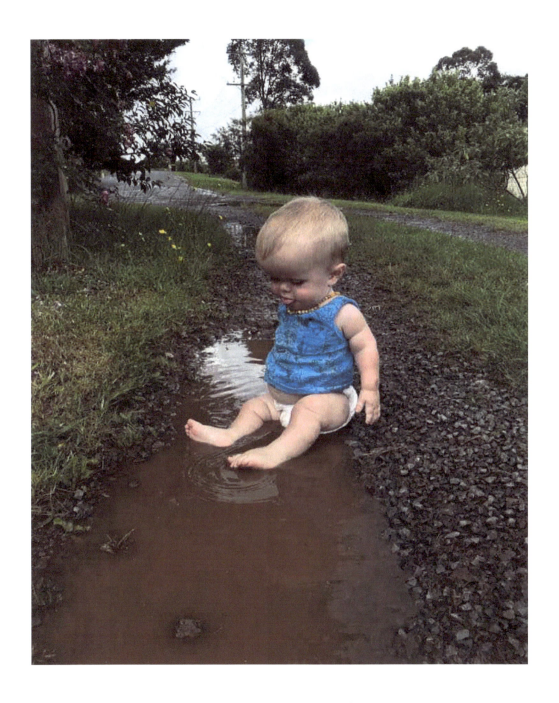

Apart from the mud
that runs through my veins,
my blood is bright red,
is yours just the same?
It's red and it's gooey
and freaks my mum out,
when I've scraped
on the wire fence,
my blood gushes out.
She fusses and kisses
and washes it clean,
til no drop of blood
can now be seen.
She offers me cupcakes
to help me forget
the pain of that fence
and the scrape I regret.

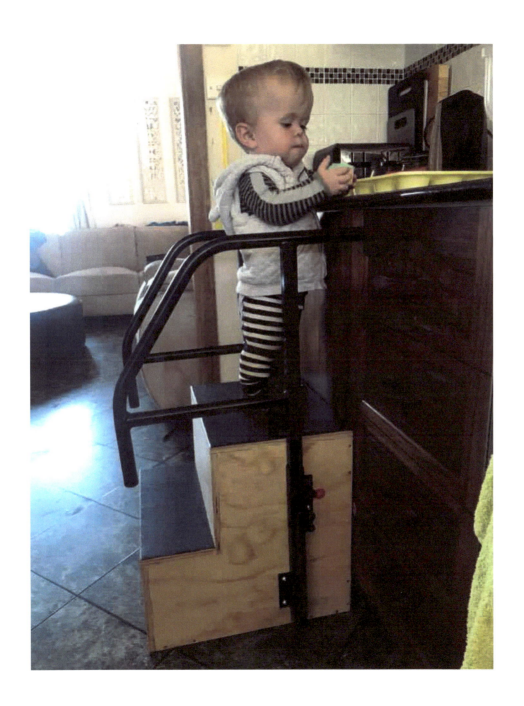

I can do all the things
that most everyone likes,
such as fishing and soccer
and riding my bike.
I play just the same
as all of my friends
and the things they don't like,
I don't like to the end.
Such as going to bed
when I'm on a roll,
or eating the broccoli
left in my bowl.
If my room is a mess,
I really don't mind
'cause my toys on the floor
are so easy to find.

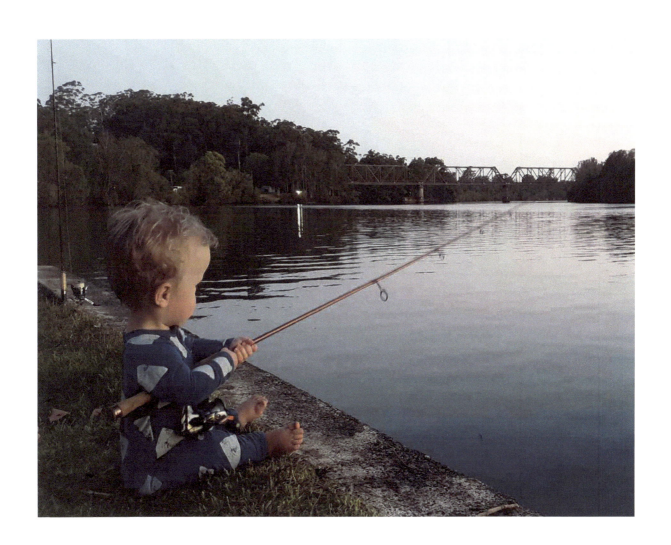

I'm strong as an ox
when I want to be.
I drive my mum nuts
when she's talking to me.
'Cause I'm far too busy,
too busy right now,
to heed all her words
as I stand on the bow
of my ship as it sails
through tempest and storm,
'cause I'm fighting dragons
that threaten to swarm.
If it wasn't for me
Mum would be dragon bait,
'cause my name is Theo,
Theo the Great.

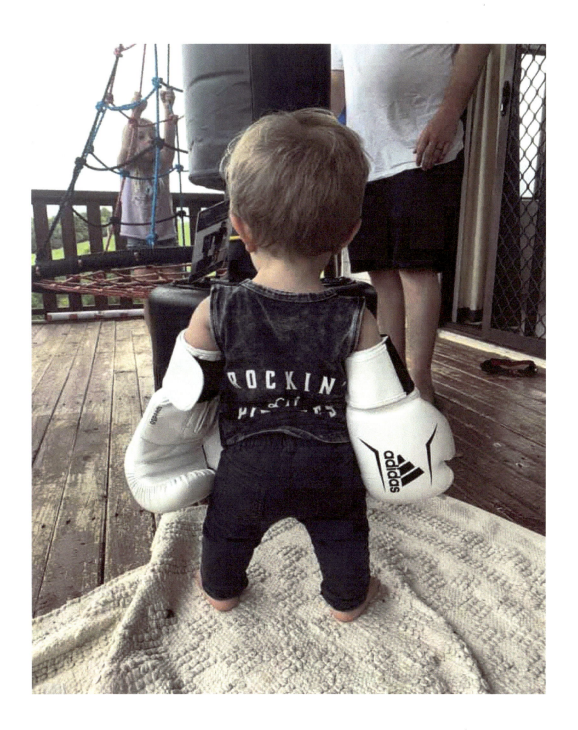

My legs may be short
but that doesn't stop me.
I march through the creek,
determined and carefree.
Some may just stare
so I'll look at them too
and smile my best smile
'cause it's just what I do.
Size is no problem,
at least not for me,
my world is so huge
with lots more to see.
I love to explore,
and figure things out
and discover new things,
of this there's no doubt.

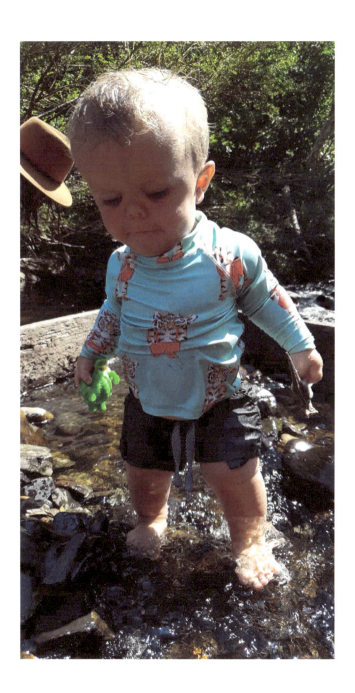

My brain's like a sponge
as it sucks up the new.
I'll never stop learning
'cause it's just what I do.
From writing and math
to science and history,
to playing with friends
and all in my family.
With the knowledge I gain
as I grow a bit more,
you just never know,
I may study law.

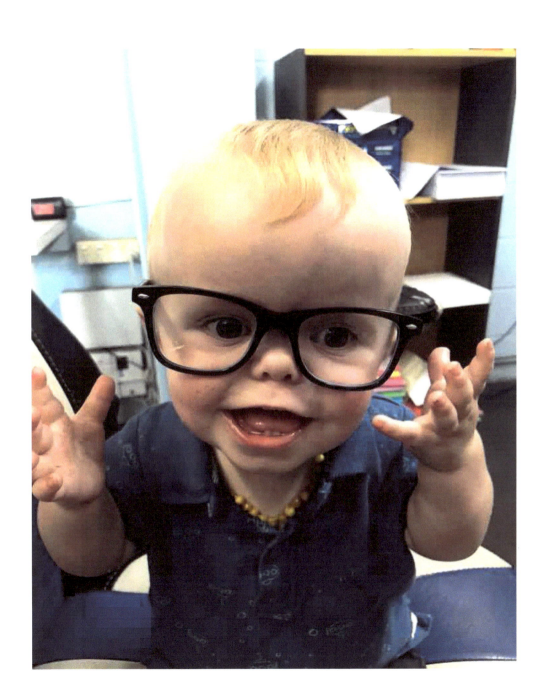

Though I live on a farm
where horses roam free,
I might be a farmer,
that sure would suit me.
I'd own lots of acres
to roam and explore,
growing fruit and potatoes
to share and adore.
But now that you know me
a little bit more,
I will not grow broccoli,
and that is for sure.
Potatoes it is,
'cause I love hot chips
and fruit is such fun
when I spit out the pips.

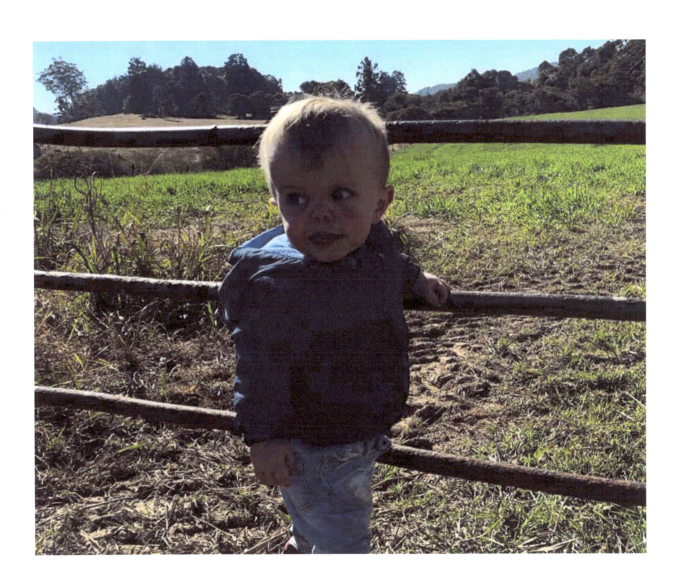

There's so much to think on,
so much to explore.
I love watching Youtube
and movies galore.
Perhaps I will be
a Director one day
and make lots of movies
and people will say,
that man may be short,
but oh goodness me,
he's the bestest Director
that we've ever seen.
I'll make movies with heroes,
and pirates and more,
and all sorts of actors
who won't make you snore.

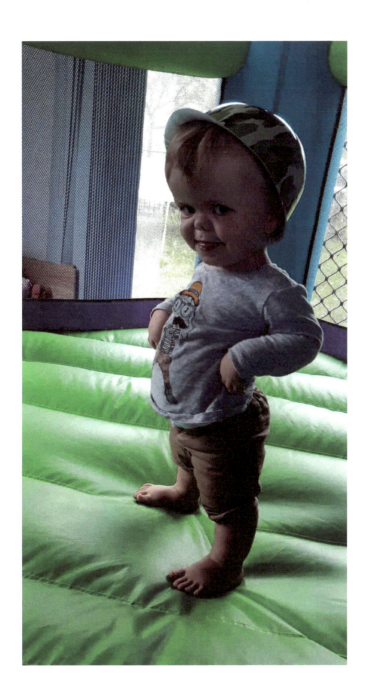

An architect sounds cool,
I could build to the sky
and ride on the elevator
way up and so high.
I would stand in my penthouse
at the upper most top,
looking down at the people
who now look like dots.
Yet it's all in my head
at this early stage,
I can't make decisions,
for it's too soon to gauge.
Right now I'm content
in my body so small
and my inside that feels
so amazingly tall.
And yet I just thought
of two other things,
and all the great wonders
that they just may bring.

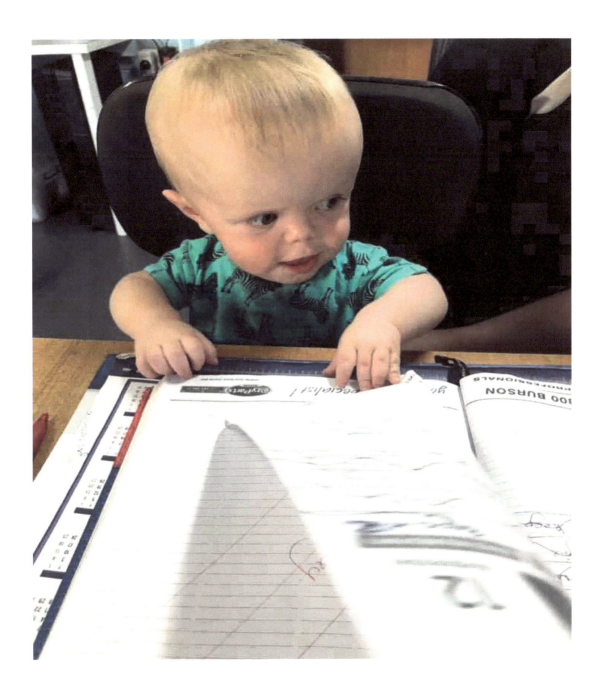

I might be a doctor
and heal all the sick,
and find what it is
that makes us all tick.
From short fat or tall
to thin as a bean,
I'm sure there'll be nothing
that I won't have seen.
Our bodies are grand
'cause guess what they do?
They carry our souls through
life's journey too.
And if you might see
one such as me,
smile and say hi
and we'll both feel quite free.

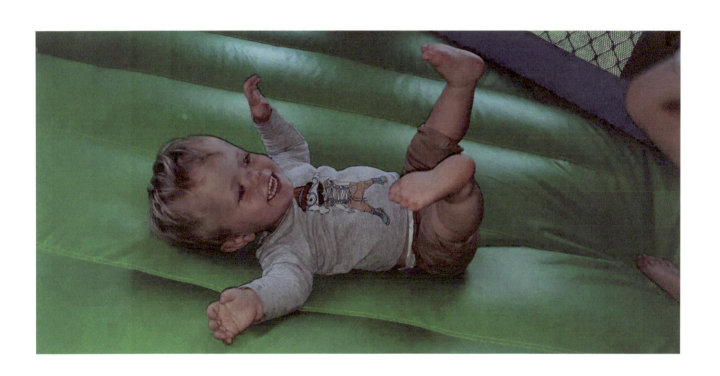

Or perhaps a great scientist
would be awesome fun.
I could have my laboratory
to observe and question.
To experiment with things
like the speed of light
and why the sun's rays
shine so hot and so bright.
Or how DNA is formed
and can change.
It's such a huge field
with such a wide range.
My brain has no limits
and I have arms and legs,
so no one will stop me,
don't bother, I beg.

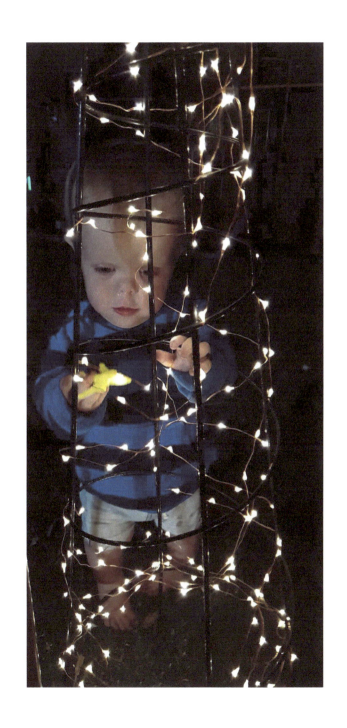

This is my sister
and she's pretty cool.
Evie's her name
and she's nobody's fool.
She's smart and she's brave
and she's bigger than me.
We have lots of fun
in this picture you'll see.
We laugh and we tussle,
she's rarely forlorn.
Especially when she's
being my unicorn.

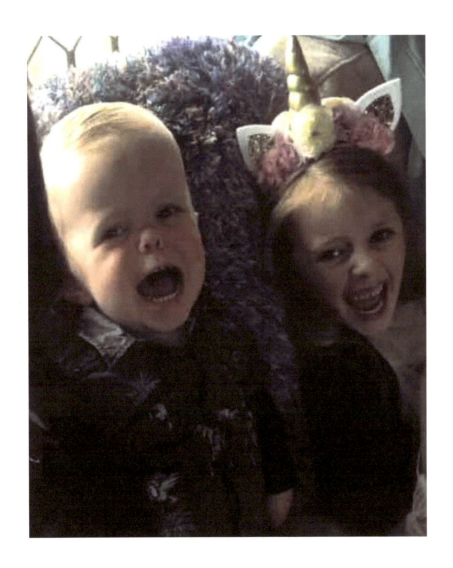

This is my hero,
he is my dad.
He's the bestest of heroes
that I've ever had.
He's brave and courageous
and tall as a tree.
He's got a tattoo
and it's all about me

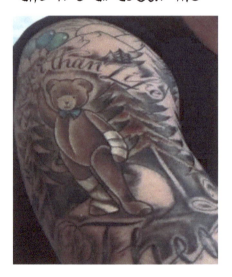

Larger than Life

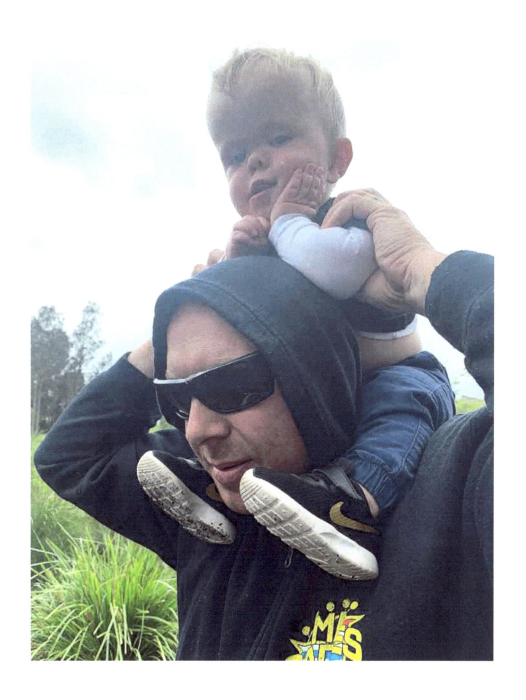

Right now I'm exhausted
as tired as can be.
My eyes, they are shut
and can no longer see.
But deep in my heart
where no one can peek,
I feel mum's love near
as she kisses my cheek.
I know that she loves me
but sometimes she'll worry
and think on the burden,
when older, I'll carry.
But this is just me
and I'll handle my fate,
so don't worry Mum
'cause I'm Theo the Great!

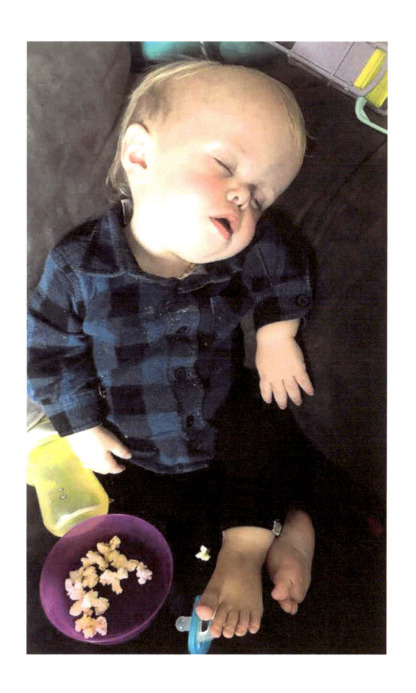

Dwarfism Life Facts

Dwarfism is so spontaneous that anyone can have a child with it. On average, 80% of babies born with dwarfism, have average height parents.

Two parents with dwarfism can have complications in having a baby.

There are over 200 types of dwarfism. The most common type being Achondroplasia.

The correct terminology for a person with dwarfism is something which is largely debated. It is best to call a person by their name, understanding that their short stature is only part of their make-up ... hence the reason we prefer to say 'a person with dwarfism'.

The word 'midget' should never be used to label or describe a person with dwarfism.

There have been many instances where sets of twins have been made of one person with dwarfism and the other being average height.

A person with dwarfism is identified as someone being 4'10" or under and having disproportionate limbs. Their torso can be average in length – depending on their dwarfism type.

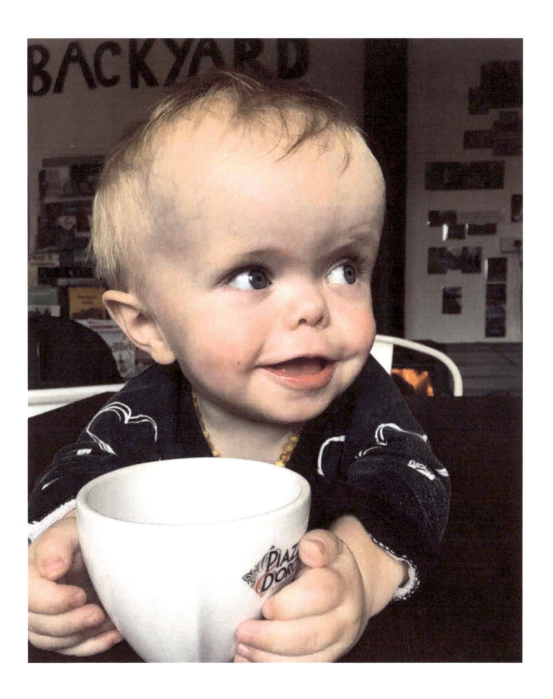

Dwarfism does not affect a person's intellectual ability. There are surgeons, teachers, professors and many other highly regarded occupations being performed by people with dwarfism.

Dwarfism is not a disease. It cannot be cured.

Most people with dwarfism would prefer a parent in public allowing their child to ask questions about the obvious difference, than to be silenced.

Just like all people, a person with dwarfism wants to be respected.

To find more information, visit Facebook.com/dwarfism4life

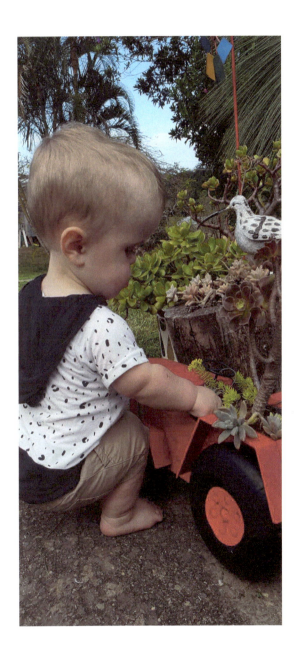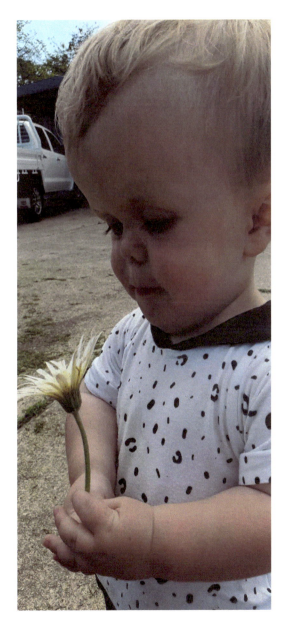

A note from Rainey Leigh Seraphine:

I would sincerely like to thank Theo and his family for allowing me the utter joy of creating a book about Theo's world.

I am honoured to live in the same community as Theo, where he is surrounded by love, respect and acceptance for the amazing little dude he is.

He may be small, but he has the hugest soul.

Without doubt, to all who know him, he is

Theo the Great!

CPSIA information can be obtained
at www.ICGtesting.com
Printed in the USA
BVHW021924080622
639278BV00006B/54